Men &

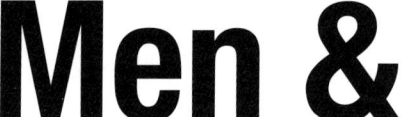

Contents

Introduction 2
Reducing your risk of cancer 4
Detecting cancer early – some DIY checks 12
Prostate cancer 14
Bowel cancer 17
Lung cancer 22
Skin cancer. 27
Testicular cancer 31

© Ian Banks 2012
Revision due February 2015

(069-12567)

Cartoons by Jim Campbell; those on pages 2, 3, 4, 12, 15, 17, 22, 27 and 31 used by kind permission of the Irish Cancer Society www.cancer.ie

ISBN: 978 0 85761 031 7

All rights reserved. No part of this booklet may be reproduced or transmitted in any form or by any means, electronic or mechanical, including photocopying, recording or by any information storage or retrieval system, without permission in writing from the copyright holder.

Printed in the UK.

Haynes Publishing, Sparkford, Yeovil, Somerset BA22 7JJ, England

Haynes North America, Inc, 861 Lawrence Drive, Newbury Park, California 91320, USA

Haynes Publishing Nordiska AB, Box 1504, 751 45 Uppsala, Sweden

The Author and the Publisher have taken care to ensure that the advice given in this edition is current at the time of publication. The Reader is advised to read and understand the instructions and information material included with all medicines recommended, and to consider carefully the appropriateness of any treatments. The Author and the Publisher will have no liability for adverse results, inappropriate or excessive use of the remedies offered in this book or their level of effectiveness in individual cases. The Author and the Publisher do not intend that this book be used as a substitute for medical advice. Advice from a medical practitioner should always be sought for any symptom or illness.

Introduction

In truth, men are more likely to look after their cars than their own bodies. Not least with regular MOT checks. Much the pity because many cancers can be prevented and most treated successfully if caught early. We need a Male MOT check and here it is for cancer. It arms you with the information you need to keep your body humming like a finely-tuned engine, so you can reduce your risk and, where possible, prevent cancer. It also gives you the tools to notice early warning signs that need to be checked out, so that little problems don't become big problems.

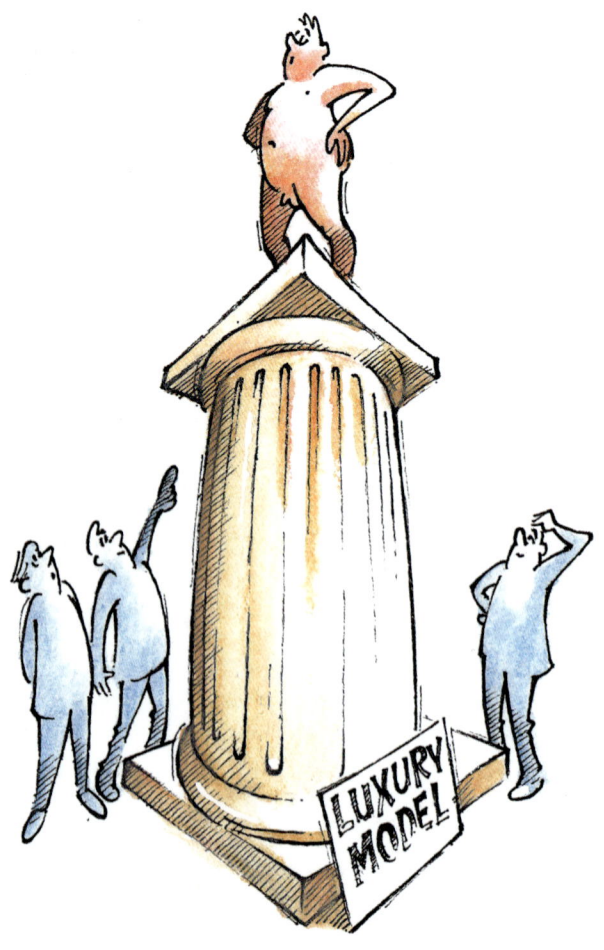

MISTER MYTHS

Remember the old myth that cars can run on water? Then they found out engines actually do work better in the rain because damp air makes the fuel burn more efficiently.

Well, cancer has its own myths and old wives' tales. It turns out that some of these myths are partly true – but others are definitely false...

Living under power lines causes cancer
Although a popular view, there is no evidence for this.

Pesticides cause cancer
A long runner this one but without good support. What we do know is there are clear links between many industrial chemicals and some cancers. So if you work with these chemicals, wear protective gear.

Mobile phones cause brain tumours
Not proven, but the monthly bills can be pretty life threatening!

Masturbation causes testicular or prostate cancer
Definitely false!

Tight underpants cause testicular cancer
False and yet falsetto.

Regularly eating burnt meat cooked on a BBQ won't increase your risk for cancer
False. Eating burnt meat regularly can increase your risk for cancer.

Men don't get breast cancer
Sadly untrue, but it is much less common in men yet the outcome is worse.

Women have prostates but they don't cause as much trouble
False. Which is great news, otherwise two people might have to get up in the middle of the night for a pee!

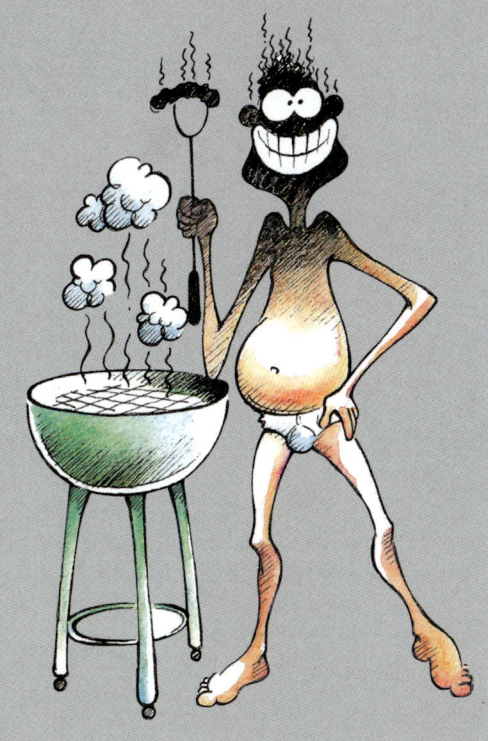

4 MEN & CANCER

Reducing your risk of cancer

WHAT ARE THE ODDS?

Your risks explained...

- Some dangers to health and life are very serious but the risk of actually suffering from them may be very small. These risks can be difficult to work out. It can also be very confusing trying to compare risks.

- For example, the risk of being killed in the UK by lightning is 1 in 10 million. This doesn't mean very much to most of us. So try thinking about it this way:

- If there was a line of people 10,000 kilometres (6,210 miles) long, only one person in the line would be killed by lightning. It would take 4 months of continuous walking to reach the end of the line.

- On the other hand, if you smoke 10 cigarettes a day, you have a 1 in 200 chance of dying earlier. You would be in a line of people only 200 metres (218 yards) long. It would take you only 4 minutes to walk from the beginning to the end.

Now it starts to make sense.

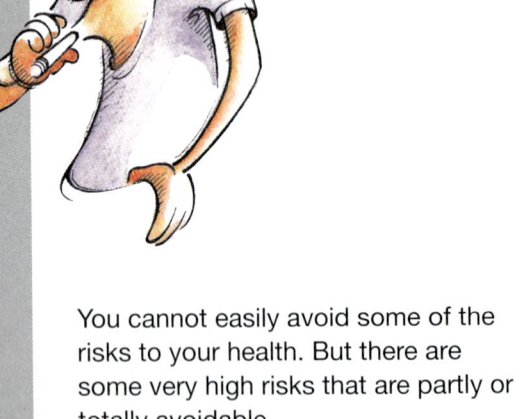

You cannot easily avoid some of the risks to your health. But there are some very high risks that are partly or totally avoidable.

Your level or risk depends on:

- What you eat.
- What you drink.
- Whether you smoke.
- How active you are.
- How you look after yourself in the sun.

MEN & CANCER 5

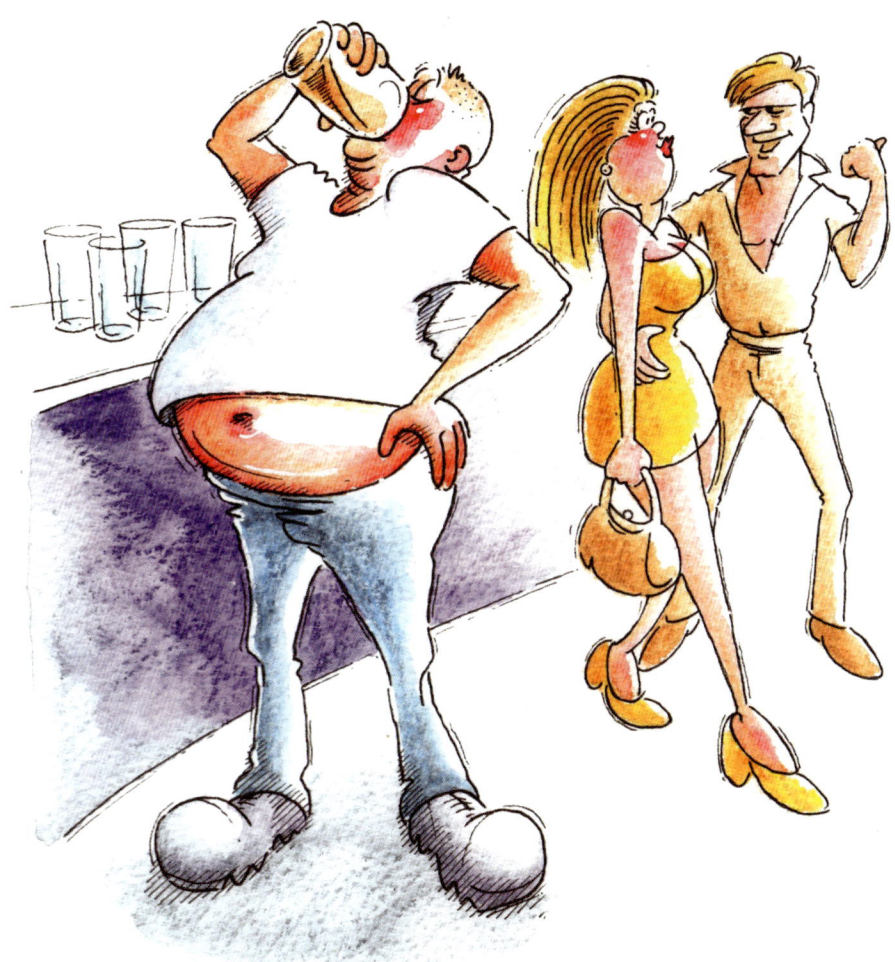

You can reduce your risk further by having regular GP check-ups; and being more aware of early signs and symptoms of ill health.

Drinking it...
The great myth is that alcohol improves performance. Not so.

How much?
Aim for no more than 3 to 4 units per day on a regular basis.

Alcohol is high in gut-adding calories, and it's linked to some cancers. The next time you're on a night out, try switching to soft drinks or non-alcoholic beers as the evening goes on – and have a few glasses of water in-between to help keep you in top gear for the whole night.

6 MEN & CANCER

The number of units of alcohol in a drink depends on the amount (volume) and strength (ABV – alcohol by volume)

- A pint of 3.5 % lager, beer or cider = 1.5 units.
- A pint of 5% lager, beer and cider = 3 units.
- A 25ml shot = 1 unit.
- A 175ml glass of wine = around 2 units.
- A 250ml glass of wine = around 3 units.
- A 25ml of spirits (a pub single) = 1 unit.
- A 5% bottle of alcopop = 1.4 units.
- A bottle of wine = around 10 units.

Know your units – www.units.nhs.uk

Eating it...

Fuel foods
Vegetables, fruits, pulses (peas and beans) and wholegrain bread, brown rice or durum wheat pasta, help keep energy flowing without piling on the weight. And as they have more nutrients and are higher in fibre, they can also protect you from cancer. The great thing is they make you feel as though you have a full tank so you're less hungry.

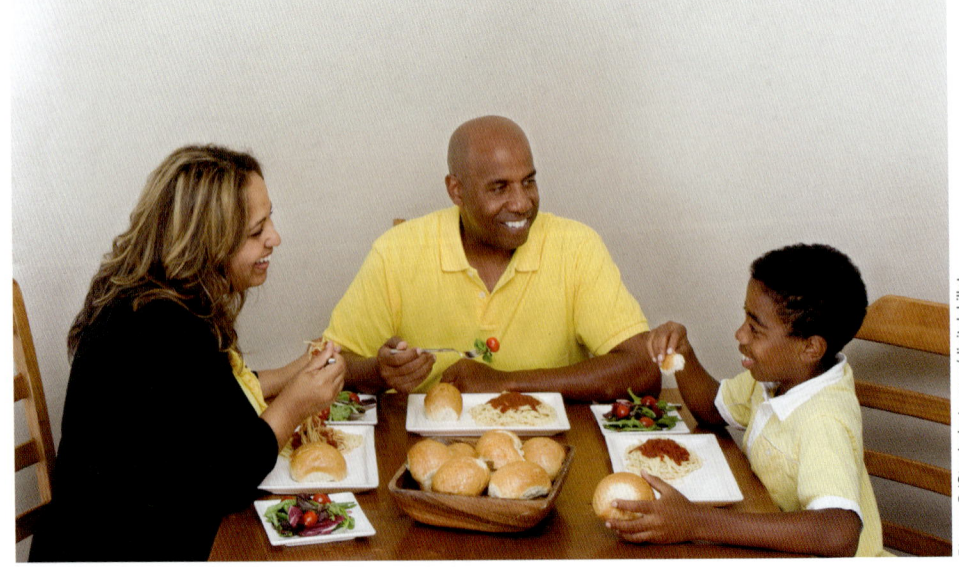

MEN & CANCER   7

It's easy to build at least

5

different fruit and veg into your day.

One portion is:

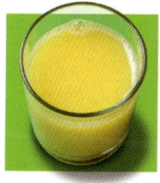
1 medium glass of orange juice

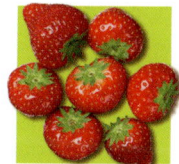
7 strawberries

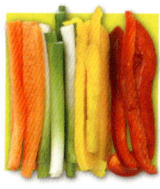
A handful of sliced peppers, onions and carrots

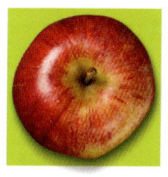
1 medium apple

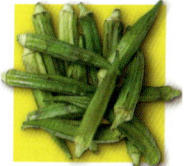
16 okra

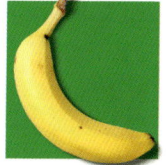
1 medium banana

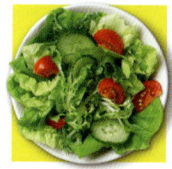
1 small mixed salad

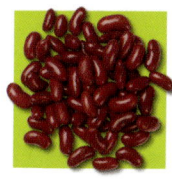
3 heaped tablespoons of cooked kidney beans

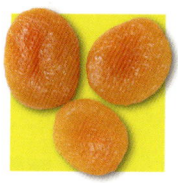
3 whole dried apricots

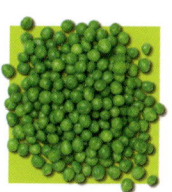
3 heaped tablespoons of peas

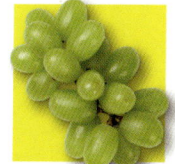
1 handful of grapes

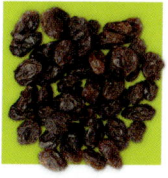
1 tablespoon raisins

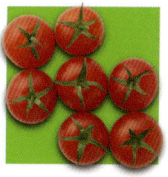
7 cherry tomatoes

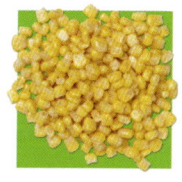
3 heaped tablespoons of corn

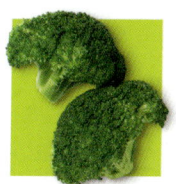
2 spears of broccoli

Carbs for your engine

Carbohydrates are the power fuel. You put your foot down and feel the push. Fats are more suited to tractors. Great for slow, heavy machinery.

So, remember fruit, vegetables and high fibre for maximum speed and energy.

Try to increase your fruit and veg to 5 or more portions a day and base your meals on high fibre bread, cereals, pasta and potatoes.

Meat and potatoes anyone?

Not a vegetarian? No problem. You don't need to miss out on the meat

BELT SIZE

If your belt size is 37 inches (92cm) or over, you are significantly increasing your risk of cancer, heart disease, diabetes and stroke. And this risk rises as your belt size goes up.

option. Like many things in life, lean meat is good for you in moderation.

Fat but fit?

Us guys eat too much fat. You can be fit and fat. But the extra fat will still cause you problems such as high

DOES WHAT IT SAYS ON THE TIN

Food labels must by law show the amount of fat.

- Avoid or cut down foods with over 20g of fat per 100g of food or over 5g of saturated fat per 100g of food.
- Aim for less than 3g of fat and under 1.5g of saturated fat per 100g of food.

www.eatwell.gov.uk/healthydiet/fss/fats/satfat

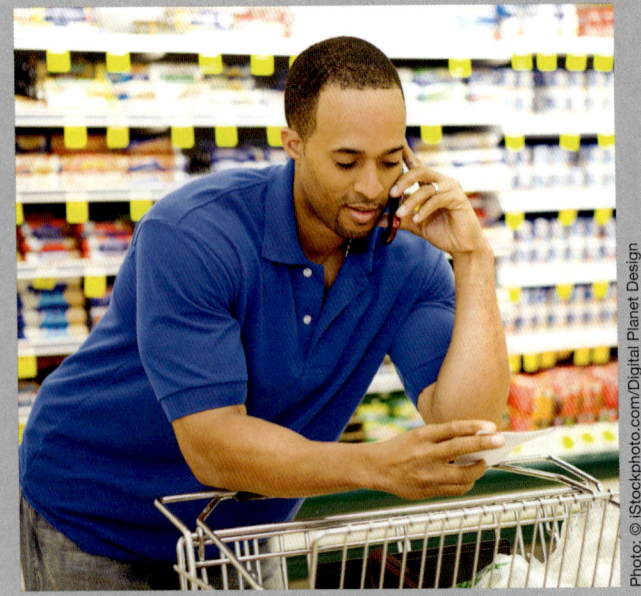

MEN & CANCER

blood pressure and heart disease. It will also increase your risk of cancer.

What's important is the mix of food on your plate. The ideal mix is one-third or less of meat, chicken or fish and two-thirds of vegetables and pasta or rice.

Fat fact
Not all fat is bad. Some fat actually helps reduce your risk of heart disease and cancer. The amount and type that we eat makes all the difference. Saturated fat clogs the fuel lines so go for unsaturated fat like olive oil.

Man on the move
A stressful life often means you eat on your feet. Not all of us have the luxury of sit down meals during the day, but this doesn't mean the upright meal has to be harmful. Takeaway foods, sausage rolls, pastries, cakes and ready-made meals often contain high levels of saturated fat and salt. For lunch have a healthy sandwich instead.

Avoid adding fat to food when you cook at home. Try not to fry. Boil, bake or grill instead.

Why watch television chefs when you can do better? Get a wok and reduce your workload. Throw in thinly sliced vegetables, some lean meat and a light coating of olive oil and serve with rice. Presto! A TV meal.

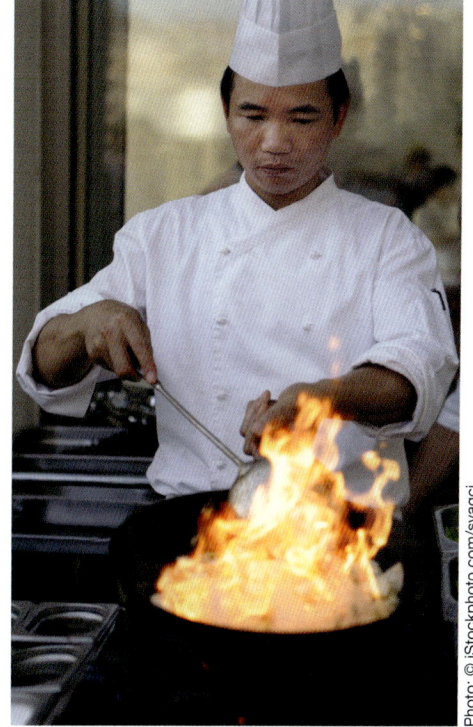

Follow up with fresh fruit in a bowl of low fat yoghurt. If you cook like this, you can get a big meal and still have plenty of change from a £5 note.

Revving it up

Getting fit doesn't mean you have to spend your time in a room full of Adonises and machines last seen in the Chamber of Horrors. Charity shops are full of fitness equipment bought by well-meaning men (or their partners) but never used.

MEN & CANCER

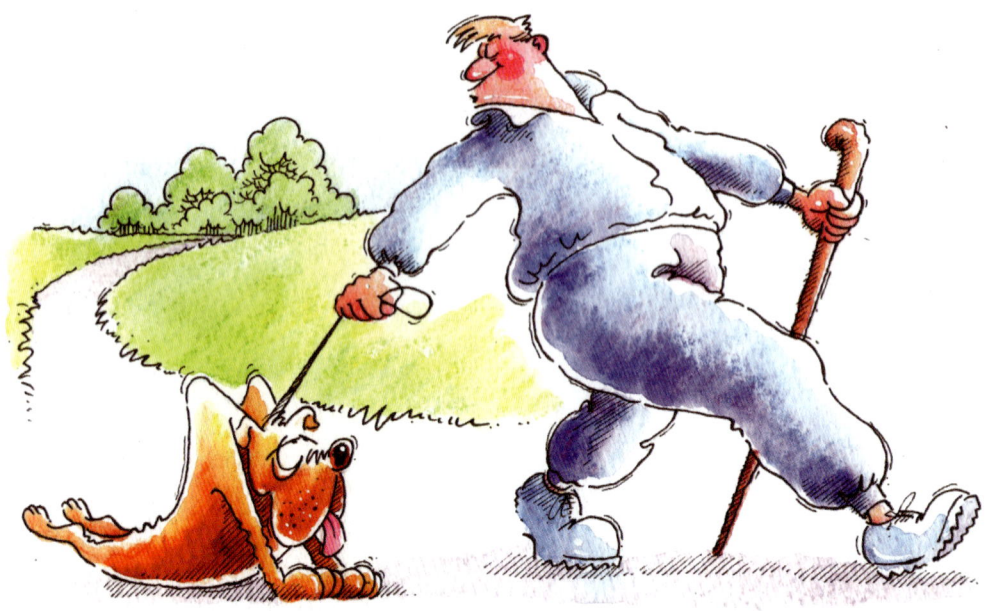

Sport is a great way of keeping fit but most of us overestimate what we need to do to stay healthy. All you need is about 30 minutes of moderate intensity physical activity most days to help reduce your risk from heart disease and some cancers.

And you don't have to do 30 minutes all in one go, activity can be accumulated throughout the day in 10 minute bouts.

All activity is of some benefit, whether at work, leisure or playing a sport. So try walking to the next bus stop and get off one stop early, use the stairs instead of the lift, walk up the escalators instead of staring at the adverts or even try some gardening (or wash the car yourself!).

Small things like these will make a big difference to your risk.

Smoking it...

Even filters won't stop this one. Smoke should leave a finely-tuned engine, not enter it. Tobacco kills more men in the world each year than WWII, murder, rival football supporters and teenage daughters' telephone bills combined!

DON'T BE FOOLED

Low tar products or filters only con you. The simple fact of the matter is that smoking kills, be it from cancer or heart disease. Not a lot of men know this but it is also one of the major causes of erectile dysfunction (often called 'impotence'). Perhaps that's why the film stars tend to smoke after the steamy love scene rather than before!

Quitting 20 cigarettes a day will save around £2,000 each year. In 5 years you could buy a half-decent car and in 10 years a nice sports model! Since the price of tobacco continues to rise, quitting could buy you a serious motor.

If you smoke, quitting is the most effective step you can take to reduce your risk of cancer – and not just lung cancer. So set a date to quit.

Burning it...

Skin cancer is on the increase and is already one of the commonest cancers in the UK. It is almost always caused by over-exposure to the sun, so protect your bodywork.

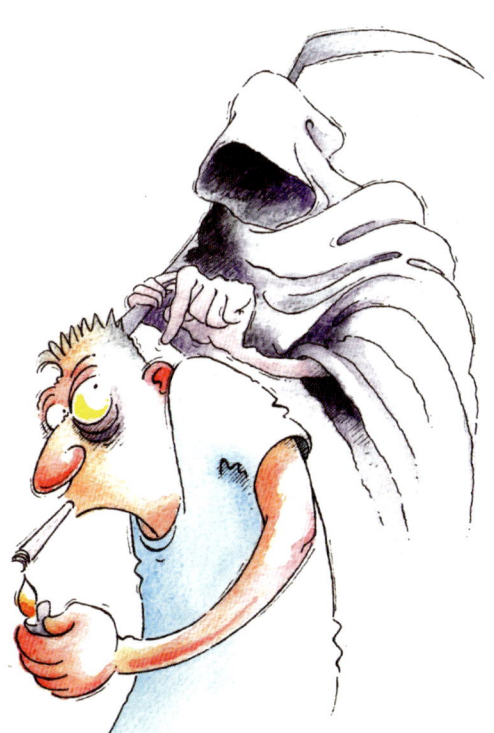

WHEN YOU STOP SMOKING . . .

. . . the benefits to your health begin straight away. As your body starts to return to normal, you will start to feel healthier, and within a few weeks you will also start to notice the benefits. For example:

- After one month – your skin will be clearer, brighter and more hydrated.

- After 3 to 9 months – your breathing will have improved, and your airways will be clearer.

- After one year – your risk of heart attack and heart disease will have fallen by half.

- After 10 years – your risk of lung cancer will have fallen by half.

- After 15 years – your risk of heart attack and heart disease is the same as someone who has never smoked.

Research into smoking shows that people who quit smoking before the age of 35 have a life expectancy only slightly less than people who have never smoked. Those who quit before they are 50 years of age reduce their risk of dying from a smoking-related disease by 50%.

12 MEN & CANCER

Detecting cancer early – some DIY checks

Keep an eye on your bodywork

The MOT check keeps your car safely on the road and can pick up faults before they become dangerous. Regular check-ups by your own GP can also pick up potential medical problems in the same way. Some GPs and wellman clinics offer tests and checkups. It's a good opportunity to talk about any concerns you might have and check out your risks.

Know what is normal for you

Get to know your toilet habits and if they change for four weeks or more, go and see your doctor.

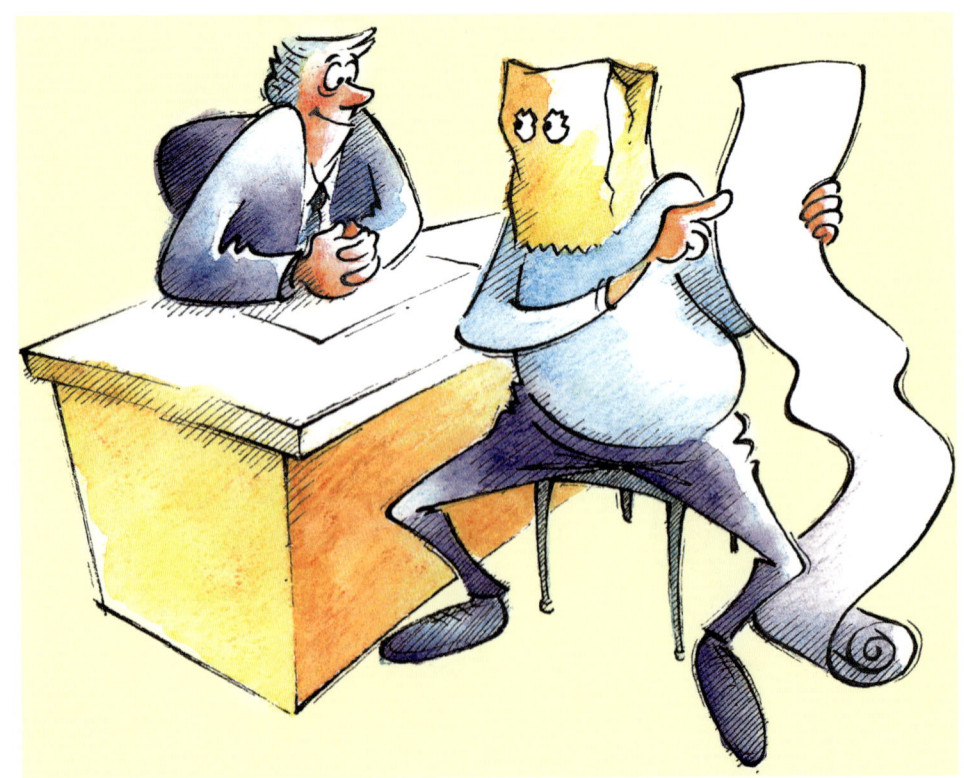

Get to know your skin so that you'll more quickly recognise anything amiss such as:

- New lumps or growths.
- A sore or bruise that does not heal.
- A mole that changes in shape, size or colour or bleeds in unusual circumstances.

Be aware of how your testicles (balls) usually feel and check them regularly for anything unusual such as a lump, thickening or swelling.

Service history

One careful driver on the logbook? Check out your family history of cancer: some cancers have a family link, especially if either of your parents suffered from a particular cancer before 60.

If you do have a parent who had cancer at an early age, check with your doctor what you can do to reduce your own risk. Your doctor may suggest regular tests, which can catch potential problems early.

Most cancers can be successfully treated when they are caught early. But remember, prevention is better than cure, so you should try to reduce your risks.

Take action if you experience any of the following for more than a couple of weeks:

- A persistent cough or hoarseness.
- Persistent indigestion or difficulty in swallowing.
- Shortness of breath.
- Significant weight loss (for no good reason).
- Loss of appetite.
- A noticeable, persistent change in bowel or bladder habits, for no good reason.

Many symptoms that might indicate cancer can also be caused by a less serious illness. But it's always better to be safe. So go see your doctor if in any doubt.

Prostate cancer

What you should know about prostate cancer...

It's exclusively a man thing. The prostate is a walnut-sized gland that sits just under the bladder. Its job is to produce the bulk of semen to help protect and nourish sperm on their hazardous trip to the womb.

What causes it?

While nobody knows what causes prostate cancer, there are some recognised risk factors:

- Birthdays: Risk increases over the age of 50 years. Prostate cancer is rare in younger men. Either buy fewer candles for the cake, or better still eat the candles and leave the cake (a high fat diet may also be a risk factor).
- Family history: If your father or brother had prostate cancer, your risk increases. If they had it at an early age, your risk is even higher. Talk to your GP.

PROSTATE PORKIES

Prostate cancer is not caused by vasectomy, injury, masturbation or reading the Kama Sutra under the bed with a torch.

- Western diet: High fat, lots of red meat. Countries with low fat and low meat diets have low levels of prostate cancer.
- Obesity: Being overweight is a major risk factor for all cancers.

Happy Birthday with many returns

As men get older, their urine flow can become slower and the bladder needs to be emptied more often, thus more trips to the loo. This is usually due to enlargement of the prostate gland putting pressure on the uretha (the tube that carries urine from the bladder to the penis). If you need to pee more often, it does not mean that you have prostate cancer. But it is important to see the doctor and rule it out. With early discovery, prostate cancer can be treated very successfully.

The symptoms of all prostate problems are similar:

- Needing to pass water (pee) often, especially at night.
- Difficulty in starting to pee.
- Straining to pee or taking a long time to finish.
- Pain when passing water or during sex when you have an orgasm.

MEN & CANCER 15

Other, less common symptoms that may be prostate cancer are:

- Pain in the lower back, hips or pelvis.
- Blood in the urine (this is unusual for prostate cancer, but may be a sign of another disease).

However, these symptoms are often due to something else and not cancer.

Prostate cancer is different from most cancers – some prostate cancers grow slowly and may not need treatment, but some grow quickly and need early treatment. When something goes wrong with the prostate it can affect a man's sex life, his long term health and, if it's prostate cancer, it may be fatal.

You do not have to put up with these symptoms just because you are getting older. If you are worried, you should go and see your doctor soon. Prostate problems can be diagnosed and treated.

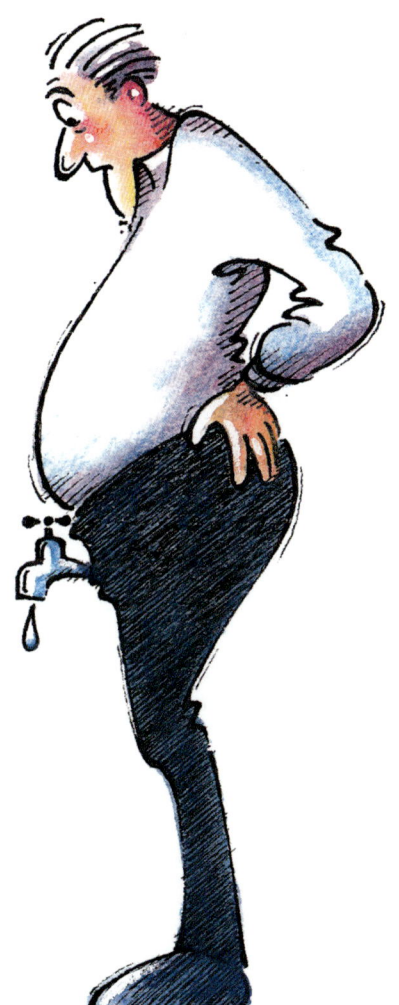

NOT A LOT OF MEN KNOW THIS

The risk of a man getting prostate cancer is only 2% less than the risk of a woman getting breast cancer.

Getting it sorted

Get used to hearing the initials 'PSA'. They stand for 'Prostate Specific Antigen' which is a simple blood test.

That's about as simple as it gets though. A raised PSA level is usually not a sign of cancer. It can be caused by inflammation and a large but non-cancerous prostate. So talk to your GP about the meaning of the results in terms of possible treatment before you consider doing a PSA test.

Your doctor will usually carry out a physical examination as well as a blood test for PSA. If the levels are high your doctor may refer you for further tests. If further tests show that you have prostate cancer, the treatment you are offered will depend on your age, general health and the stage or grade of the cancer.

For more information on the Prostate Cancer Risk Management Programme go to: www.cancerscreening.nhs.uk/prostate

Top treatments
Possible treatments include surgery, radiotherapy, hormone therapy and sometimes chemotherapy. There have been significant improvements in treatment over the past decade.

REDUCE YOUR RISK

You may be able to reduce your risk by having a balanced diet with fresh fruit and vegetables.

Tomatoes and tomato-based products reportedly can reduce your risk, so the occasional Bloody Mary may also be helpful, but preferably with less Mary!

Where can I find out more?

NHS Direct
24 hour phone line: 0845 46 47
www.nhsdirect.nhs.uk

NHS Choices
www.nhs.uk

Orchid Cancer Appeal
www.orchid-cancer.org.uk

The Prostate Cancer Charity
www.prostate-cancer.org.uk

UK Prostate Link
www.prostate-link.org.uk

MEN & CANCER

Bowel cancer

What you should know about bowel cancer...

THE SHORT AND TALL OF IT

- Bowel cancer is a disease of the large bowel (colon) or rectum. It is also sometimes called colorectal or colon cancer.
- It is the second largest cause of cancer deaths in the UK.
- In 2006 there were over 30,000 new cases of bowel cancer in England and over 14,000 deaths.
- Around one in 20 people will get bowel cancer at some point in their life.

The bowel is sometimes called the gut. It digests and absorbs food. There are two parts, the small and large bowel, which reflect the width of the gut rather than its length.

Cancer more commonly appears in the large bowel and rectum, which is the very last part of the gut. Bowel cancer is common, preventable to a degree and very treatable when caught early.

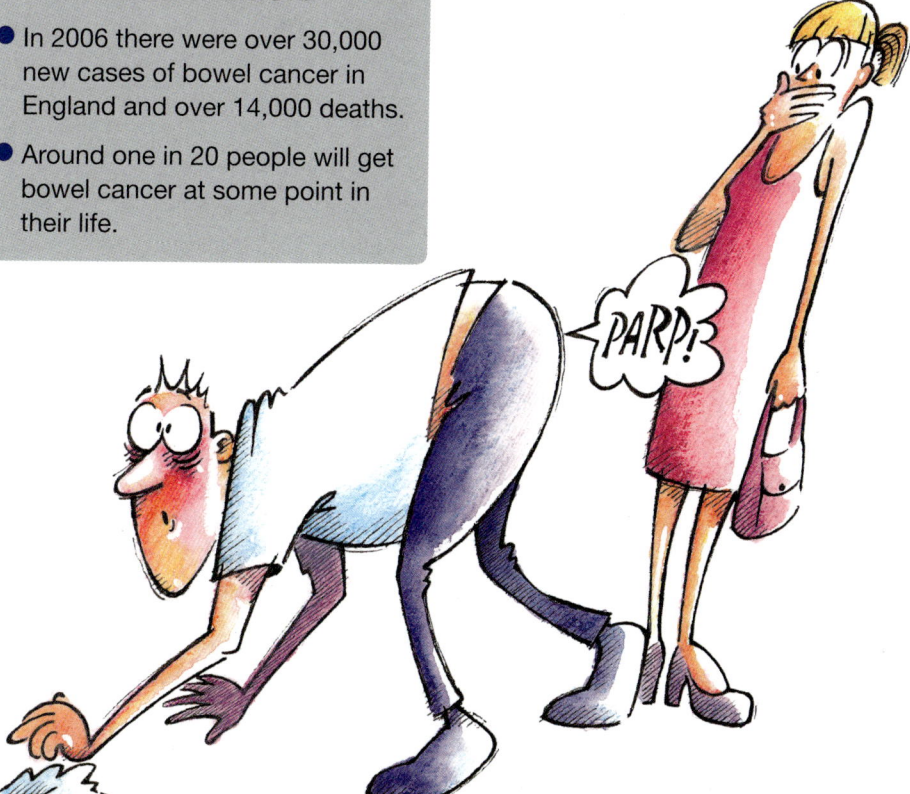

Causes of bowel cancer

The definite cause of bowel cancer is still a mystery. But we know some things do increase your risk. Your risk is higher if:

- You eat lots of junk food, fat and sugar and not enough fibre.
- Someone in your close family had bowel cancer.
- You don't exercise.
- You're overweight.
- You smoke tobacco.
- You or a member of your family have a bowel condition called polyps or adenomatous polyposis. This can significantly increase your risk. Trying to pronounce it can be pretty stressful too!

The good news is you can reduce your risk, even if bowel cancer is in the family.

- Check out your diet. Reduce the amount of fat and sugars and eat more fruit, vegetables and fibre.
- Keep your weight under control.
- Discuss your family history with your doctor, who may advise more frequent tests.
- Quit smoking.

Better sooner than later

Being 'bowel aware' is the name of the game. Guts play up at the best of times but there are some warning signs that you shouldn't ignore.

Remember! These symptoms don't always mean cancer. But if you have any of them, get your doctor to check them out.

What are the signs and symptoms of bowel cancer?

Not all bowel cancer patients will have symptoms and the symptoms may vary. Symptoms that might be bowel cancer include:

- A *persistent* change in normal bowel habit, such as going more often and diarrhoea, especially if you are also bleeding from your bottom.
- Bleeding from the bottom without any reason, particularly over the age of 50.
- A lump in your tummy or back passage felt by your doctor.
- Pain that affects your appetite.
- Unexplained iron deficiency in men or in women after the menopause.
- Unexplained weight loss.
- Unexplained extreme tiredness.

MEN & CANCER   19

- If you have any of these symptoms for four weeks you should go and see your GP.

Please remember that most of these symptoms will not be cancer.

Medical checks and treatment

Men die of embarrassment every single day in the UK. Yes, having a rectal examination is not everyone's idea of a good day out but it can save your life. It is not painful and your doctor does them every day.

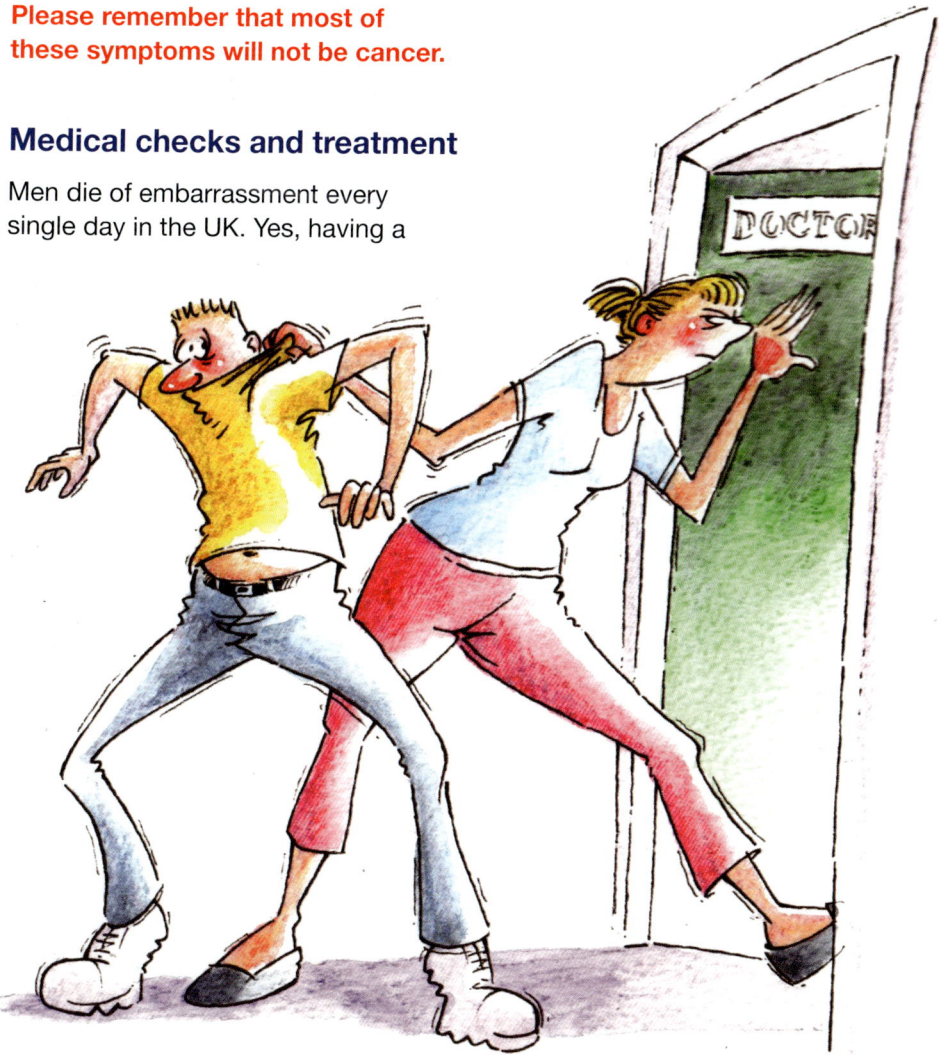

20 MEN & CANCER

THE NHS BOWEL CANCER SCREENING PROGRAMME

The NHS Bowel Cancer Screening Programme is being rolled out across England by December 2009. Men and women aged 60 to 69 are sent a testing kit to complete in the privacy of their own homes. The completed kit is sent off to a laboratory. The test is looking for hidden blood in the stools, which could mean bowel cancer. 2 out of 100 people who take the test have a positive result, and are invited to go for a bowel scope (colonoscopy) at a local screening unit.

If the programme is already operating in your area, make the decision to complete the kit when you are sent one. Research has shown that screening can cut the death rate from bowel cancer by 16% in those screened. The programme will be extended to men and women aged 70 to 75 from 2010.

Getting it sorted

If you do have bowel cancer, treatment will depend on where the cancer is, whether it has spread and your general health. Surgery is the main form of treatment, but more doctors are combining it with chemotherapy and radiotherapy.

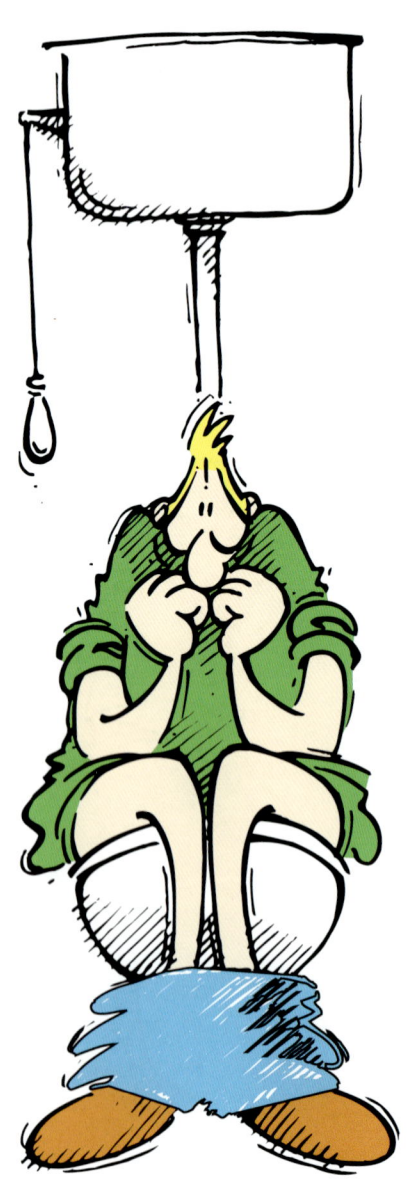

Where can I get further information?

NHS Direct
24 hour phone line: 0845 46 47
www.nhsdirect.nhs.uk

NHS Choices
www.nhs.uk

NHS Cancer Screening Programmes
www.cancerscreening.nhs.uk

Beating Bowel Cancer
www.beatingbowelcancer.org

Bowel Cancer UK
Helpline: 08708 50 60 50
www.bowelcanceruk.org.uk

Cancer Research UK
0800 226 237
www.cancerhelp.org.uk

Men's Health Forum
www.malehealth.co.uk

Lung cancer

What you should know about lung cancer...

The smoking gun

It's not difficult to work out what causes lung cancer. If you don't smoke your chances of getting it are small.

- Start early, die early. The amount of tobacco you smoke moves you that bit closer to the great scrap-yard in the sky.
- Filters and low tar don't protect you. Wise up and stub it out.
- So should you go for pipes and cigars? No way, they just give you a feeling of false security. Smoking causes cancer.
- Cut down then? That doesn't work either. You gradually creep back up. Stop completely.
- All over the country men are getting the message. That's why lung cancer in men is on the decrease. You can be one of them.

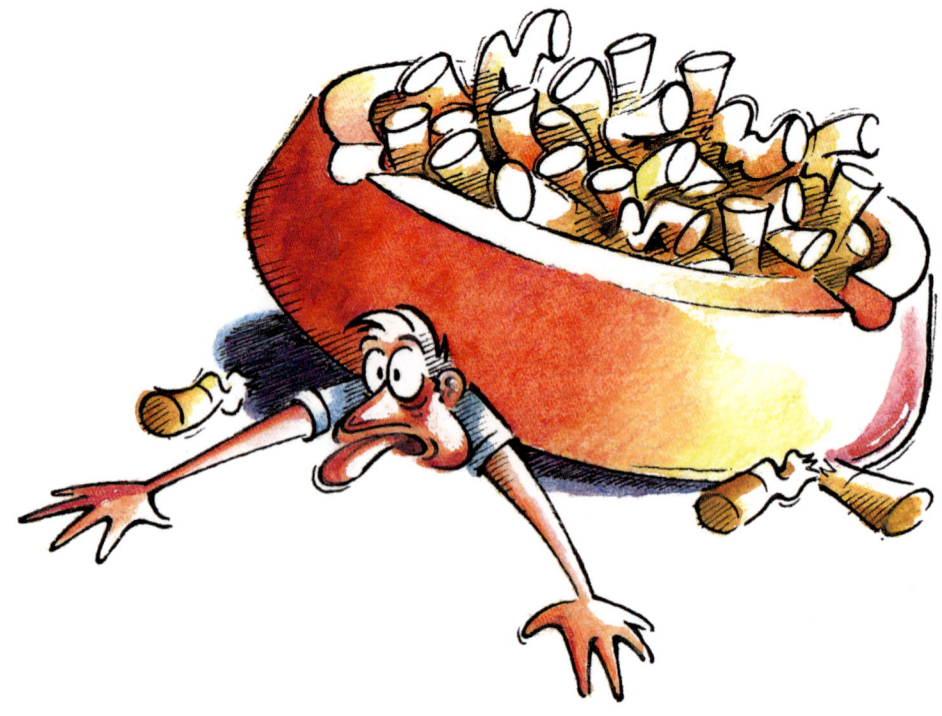

MEN & CANCER 23

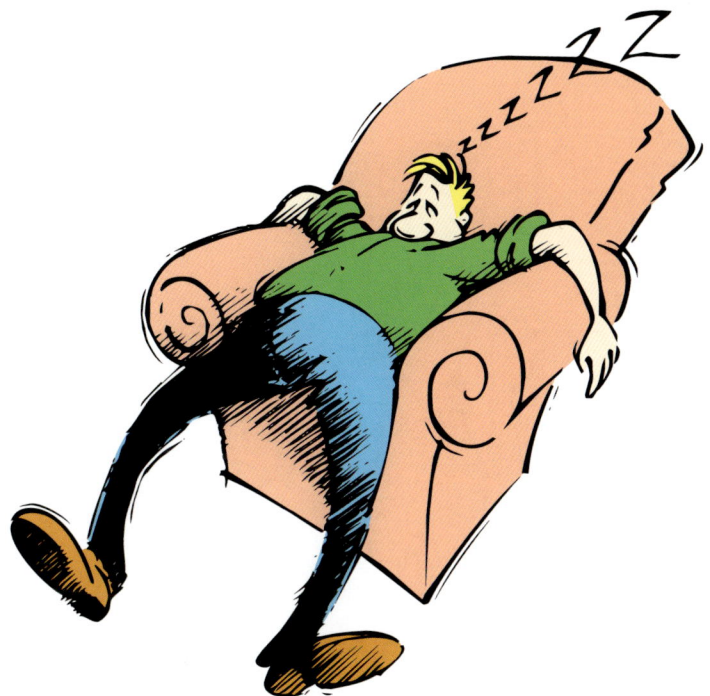

Early signs

Common symptoms of lung cancer include:

- A cough that doesn't go away after two to three weeks.
- Worsening or change of a long-standing cough.
- Persistent chest infections.
- Coughing blood.
- Unexplained persistent breathlessness.
- Unexplained persistent tiredness or lack of energy.
- Unexplained persistent weight loss.
- Persistent chest and/or shoulder pain.

There are many other causes of these symptoms, so just because you have some of them it does not mean you have lung cancer. However, these symptoms might mean something is wrong with your body. You should seek medical advice if you are concerned.

If you have a long term chest complaint such as bronchitis you should see your GP regularly as there is a link with lung cancer.

24 MEN & CANCER

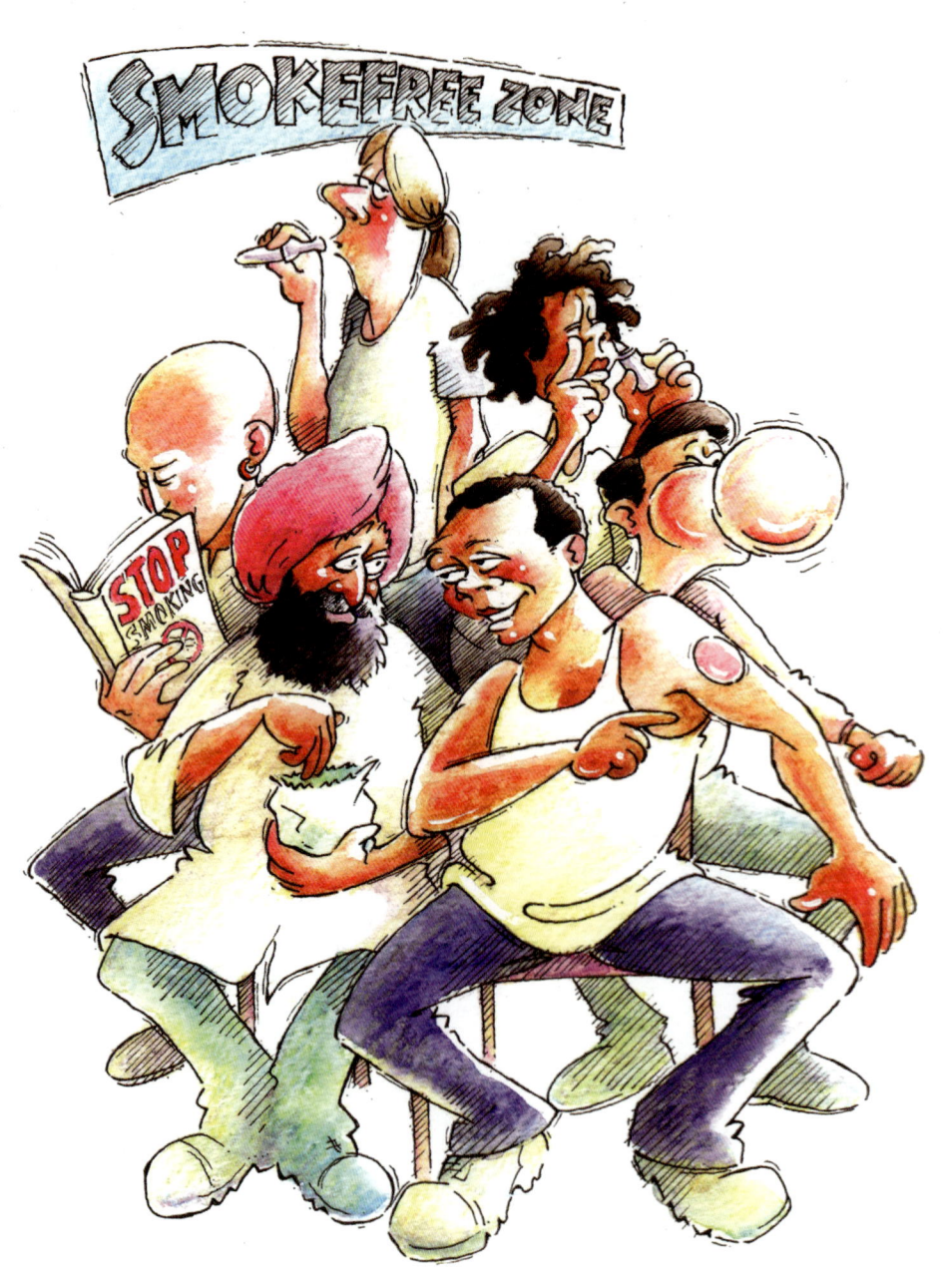

NEWS FLASH

First the good news: Lung cancer in men is preventable and on the decrease. It is almost entirely caused by smoking.
Now the bad news: Some men think they are immune…

If you have lung cancer, treatment depends on the type of cancer, how developed it is and your general state of health. Surgery, radiotherapy and chemotherapy may be used alone or together to treat lung cancer.

WAYS TO STOP

- Nicotine Replacement Therapy (NRT) can be obtained through your GP or bought over the counter in the pharmacy. Used correctly, it can be very successful in easing the cravings for nicotine. There are many types so make sure you discuss with your GP or pharmacist the best one for you.
- Get in touch with self-help groups or organisations that supply information and support.
- Ask your GP for advice on other methods that may help you quit.
- If you can't stop for yourself, do it for your partner or kids.

Remember! Early detection of lung cancer can make a difference in your chances of survival. If you have any of the symptoms listed above, see your doctor. Better still, reduce your risks of getting lung cancer by stopping smoking.

Quit plan

- List your reasons for quitting.
- Set a day and date to stop. Tell all your friends and relatives, they will support you.
- Get someone to quit with you. You will reinforce each other's willpower.
- Clear the house and your pockets of any packets, papers or matches.
- Map out your progress on a chart or calendar. Keep the money you save in a separate container.

If you get a craving, practice the 4 D's:

- Drink water; Deep breathe; Distract yourself; and Delay grabbing for that smoke for 3 minutes (cravings can take this long to disappear).
- Ask your friends not to smoke around you. People accept this far more readily than they used to do.

Where can I get more information?

NHS Direct On-line
www.nhsdirect.nhs.uk

The British Lung Foundation
08458 50 50 20
www.lunguk.org

Cancer Research UK
0800 226 237
www.cancerhelp.org.uk

Macmillan Cancer Support
0808 808 2020
www.macmillan.org.uk

Men's Health Forum
www.malehealth.co.uk

The Roy Castle Lung Cancer Foundation
Helpline: 0800 358 7200
www.roycastle.org

MEN & CANCER   27

Skin cancer

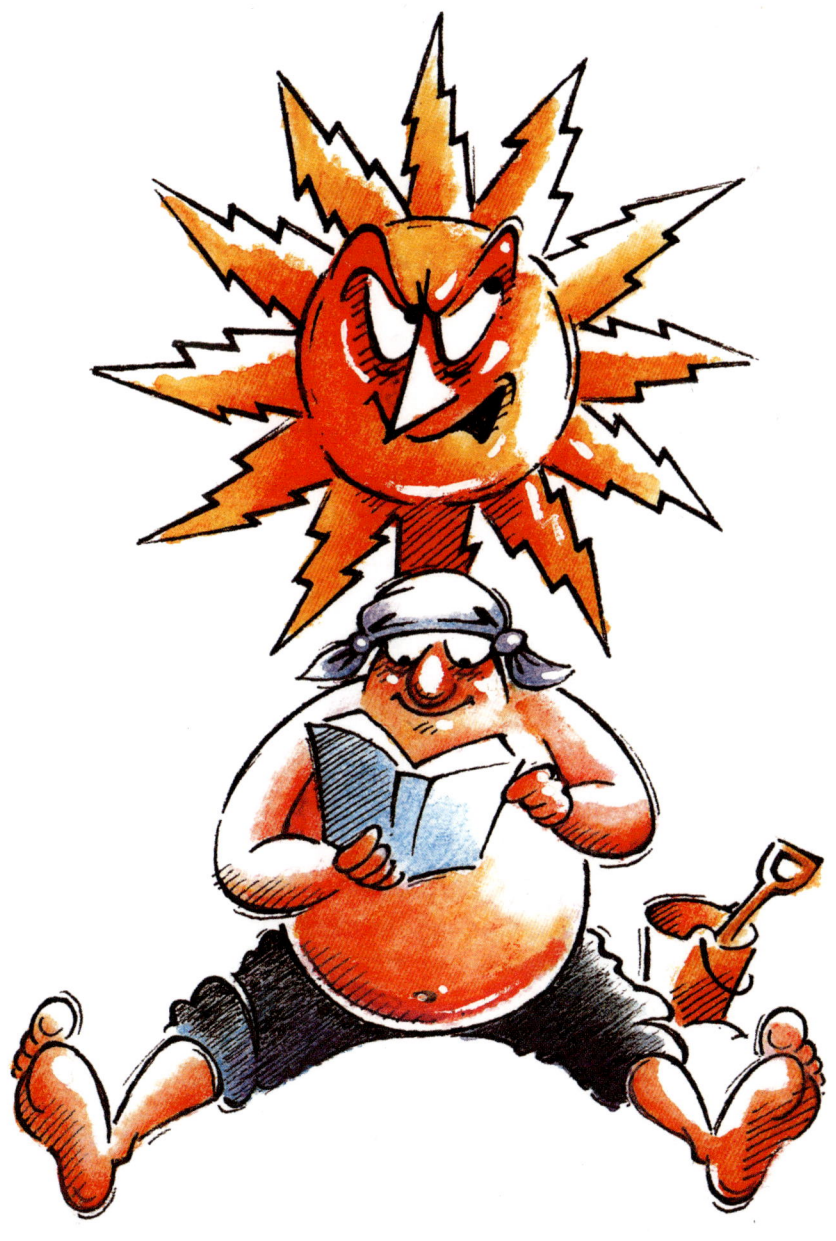

What you should know about skin cancer...

Sun sense

The sun damages your bodywork by its Ultraviolet Radiation (UV).

UV radiation causes early aging, burning and skin cancer. UVB radiation is responsible for most of this damage.

Tanning is a sign that damaged skin is trying to protect itself from the sun's ultraviolet rays.

There are basically two types of skin cancer:

- Non-melanoma is the most common form of skin cancer. It's commonly found on the forehead, tip of the chin, nose, ears, forearms and hands – basically, all the exposed bits.

- Malignant Melanoma is the more serious form of skin cancer. Although it is much less common, it is on the increase. It often appears as a changing mole or freckle but it can also develop from normal-looking skin.

Watch out for

- Size: bigger than the butt end of a pencil (more than 6 mm/quarter inch diameter).
- Colour variety: shades of tan, brown black and sometimes red or white.
- Shape: ragged or scalloped edge and one half unlike the other.
- Itchiness or bleeding.

Also watch out for

- A new growth or sore that does not heal within four weeks.
- A spot or sore that continues to itch, hurt, crust, scab or bleed.
- Constant skin ulcers that are not explained by other causes.

But skin cancer doesn't always have these features. Check your skin and moles regularly and watch out for any changes. Many skin changes are harmless but a quick check with your doctor or pharmacist can save your skin as skin cancer is much easier to treat when it is caught early.

MEN & CANCER 29

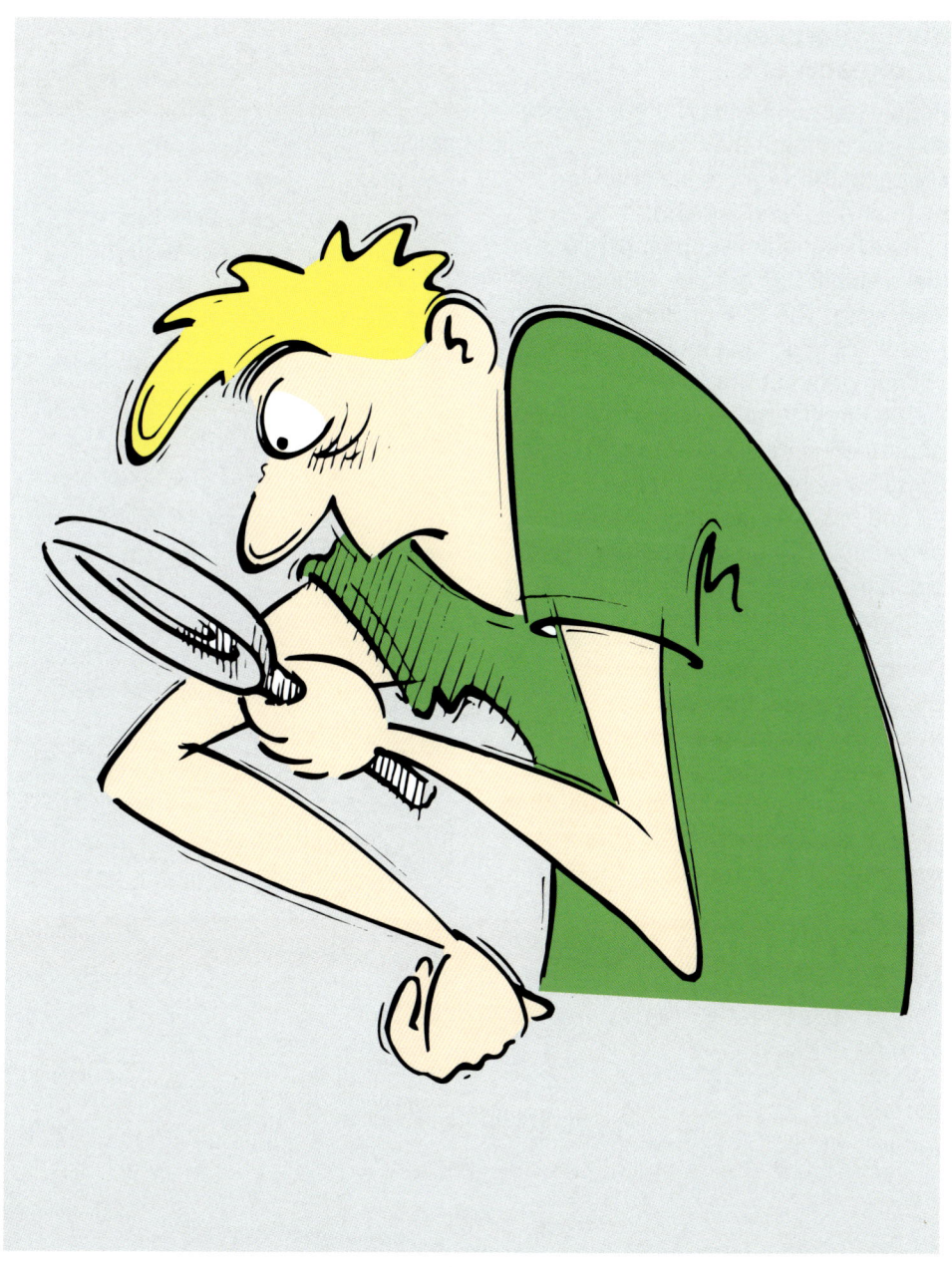

Sunscreens and smokescreens

People get confused over sunscreens and can damage their skin by choosing the wrong sunscreen for them or not using enough.

Read your sunscreen label and make sure it has both an SPF and a star rating. The SPF or Sun Protection Factor tells you how much protection you are getting from UVB rays.

The star **** rating shows the level of protection against UVA rays. Try to buy a sunscreen that is at least SPF 15 and has a 4 star rating. Apply it generously half an hour before you go out in the sun and remember to take it with you so you can reapply regularly.

Remember! Wearing sunscreen does not mean that you can stay out in the sun longer. Sunscreen offers some protection, but use it alongside covering up and spending time in the shade to give your skin the protection it needs.

NOT A LOT OF PEOPLE KNOW THIS

- Skin cancer is one of the most common cancers in the UK. And it kills more men than women (988 men to 837 women in 2007, according to the Office for National Statistics).
- Even cloudy days can deliver 90% of the dangerous UV rays.
- Some football shirts are so thin they let almost all the sunshine through.
- Skin damage remains after your sunburn fades. It builds up under the skin just like rust under bodywork paint and it can come back to haunt you in later years.
- Virtually all the risk comes from overexposure to the sun and sunbeds...

So cover up and close up!

BE SUNSMART

S pend time in the shade between 11 and 3.

M ake sure you never burn.

A im to cover up with a t-shirt, hat and sunglasses.

R emember to take extra care with children.

T hen use factor 15+ sunscreen.

MEN & CANCER 31

Testicular cancer

What you should know about testicular cancer...

The good news is testicular cancer is highly treatable. Most men who get it are cured. The bad news is it's the most common cancer in young men between 15 and 34 years in the UK. If you had an undescended testicle, your risk is significantly higher. You also have a higher risk if your father or brother suffered from testicular cancer.

It's in your hands

Be aware of how your balls normally feel by checking them on a regular but not too often basis: Be Ball Aware but not Totally Testicle.

- Cradle your scrotum in both hands using fingers and thumbs to examine and compare your testicles. Small differences in size are normal.

- Testicles should feel smooth, with no lumps, swellings or hardening present.

- There is a soft rubbery tube at the top and back of both testicles. This is called the epididymis. It carries sperm to the penis. It can be tender and it wobbles. Lumps tend to be firmly fixed to the testicle.

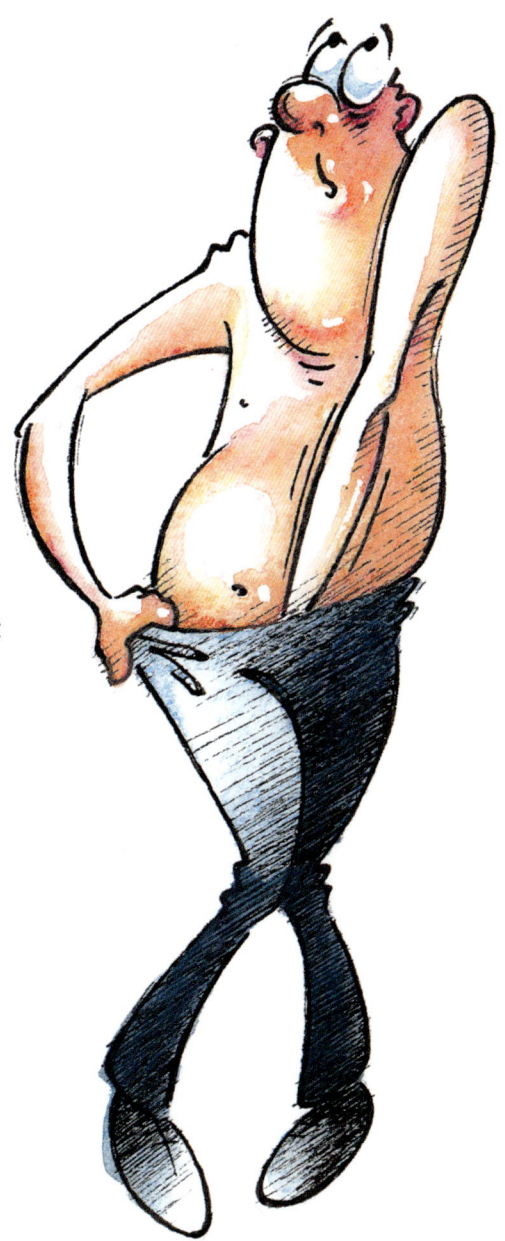

32 MEN & CANCER

You should see your doctor if:

- You can feel a small lump or swelling in either ball.
- You notice any hardening of the testicle.
- You can feel a sensation of dragging or heaviness in your scrotum.
- You experience dull aches in the groin.
- You notice any smelly pus or blood in your semen.

Thankfully, most lumps aren't cancer. But don't ignore a lump – let your doctor decide whether you need further tests. There is a range of options for treatment. Surgery, radiotherapy and chemotherapy may be used alone or together. All are highly effective. After treatment most men can have children and a normal sex life.

It's normal for one testicle to be lower than the other. It's nature's way of allowing you to cross your legs without screaming.

ON YOUR BIKE

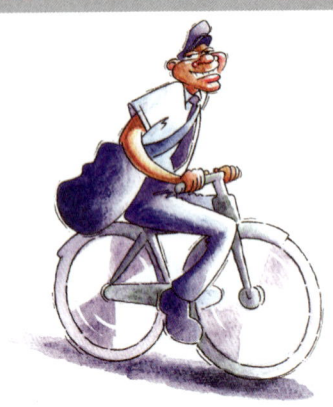

Like any injury, slipping onto the crossbar of your bike doesn't increase your risk of testicular cancer – but it might extend your vocabulary.

Where can I get further information?

NHS Direct
24 hour phone line: 0845 46 47
www.nhsdirect.nhs.uk

NHS Choices
www.nhs.uk

Orchid Cancer Appeal
www.orchid-cancer.org.uk